THE FIGHT AGAINST CANCER 2:

Foods That Prevent Cancer.

Dr. Bobby Franklin.

DEDICATION

This book is dedicated to people battling cancer and to those who have died from this deadly illness. My thoughts are with their families and loved ones. Together we can win this battle against cancer.

TABLE OF CONTENT

INTRODUCTION

While there is no surefire strategy to prevent cancer merely via dietary choices, a balanced and nutritious diet may help to decrease the risk of getting some forms of cancer. Here are some dietary tips that may help minimize the risk:

Eat A Plant-based Diet: Consume lots of fruits, vegetables, whole grains, legumes, and nuts. These foods are rich in antioxidants, fiber, vitamins, and minerals that may help protect against many malignancies.

Include Colorful Fruits And Vegetables: Aim for a range of colorful produce such as berries, leafy greens, cruciferous vegetables (e.g., broccoli, cauliflower), carrots, tomatoes, and citrus fruits. distinct hues generally signify distinct useful chemicals.

Limit Processed Foods And Red Meat: Processed meats including bacon, sausages, hot dogs, and deli meats have been related to an increased risk of colorectal cancer. Limit their consumption. Choose lean sources of protein like chicken, fish, or plant-based alternatives.

Choose Healthy Cooking Methods: Opt for steaming, baking, grilling, or sautéing instead of deep-frying or charbroiling, since high-temperature cooking techniques may release carcinogenic chemicals.

Reduce Saturated Fats And Trans Fats: Minimize the consumption of saturated fats found in fatty meats, full-fat dairy products, and fried meals. Avoid trans fats frequently found in processed snacks, baked products, and margarine.

Increase Fiber Intake: Include fiber-rich foods including whole grains, legumes, fruits, and vegetables. High-fiber diets have been related to a lower incidence of colorectal cancer.

Consume Omega-3 Fatty Acids: Omega-3 fatty acids, found in fatty fish (e.g., salmon, mackerel) and some nuts and seeds (e.g., flaxseeds, chia seeds), have anti-inflammatory characteristics that may be protective against certain malignancies.

Moderate Alcohol Intake: Excessive alcohol drinking has been related to an increased risk of numerous forms of cancer. If you wish to drink, do so in moderation (up to one drink per day for women and up to two drinks per day for males).

Limit Sugary Meals And Drinks: Diets high in added sugars may promote obesity, which is a risk factor for some cancers. Minimize the use of sugary snacks, drinks, and processed meals.

Stay Hydrated: Drink lots of water throughout the day to maintain optimum hydration and promote overall health.

Remember, keeping a healthy lifestyle extends beyond nutrition alone. Regular physical exercise, keeping a healthy weight, avoiding cigarettes and excessive sun exposure, getting adequate sleep, managing stress, and regular checkups are all beneficial for minimizing cancer risk.

HOW DOES FOOD PREVENT CANCER

Certain foods and dietary habits may have a role in lowering the risk of cancer. While no one meal will ensure the prevention of cancer, a balanced diet consisting of many healthful foods may contribute to general health and perhaps lessen the chance of getting certain forms of cancer. Here are several ways in which diet might aid in cancer prevention:

Antioxidants: Many fruits, vegetables, and whole grains are rich in antioxidants, which help protect cells from harm caused by free radicals. Free radicals are unstable chemicals that may damage DNA and other biological components, possibly leading to cancer. Examples of antioxidant-rich foods include berries, leafy greens, tomatoes, and almonds.

Phytochemicals: Phytochemicals are naturally occurring molecules found in plants that have been related to a decreased risk of cancer. These chemicals have diverse protective effects, such as decreasing inflammation, preventing carcinogens, and slowing the formation of cancer cells. Foods high in phytochemicals include cruciferous vegetables (e.g., broccoli, cabbage), garlic, soybeans, and green tea.

Fiber: High-fiber meals, such as whole grains, legumes, fruits, and vegetables, may assist in keeping a healthy digestive tract. Fiber helps to regulate bowel motions, stimulates the evacuation of waste and toxins from the body, and lowers the time that potentially dangerous chemicals spend in the digestive system. This may help lessen the risk of colorectal cancer.

Healthy Fats: Including sources of healthy fats in the diet, such as avocados, nuts, seeds, and fatty fish (high in omega-3 fatty acids), may be advantageous. These fats have anti-inflammatory characteristics and may help lower the incidence of some malignancies, including breast and colorectal cancer.

Reduced Processed And Red Meat Consumption: Consuming excessive quantities of processed meats (e.g., sausages, bacon) and red meats (e.g., beef, hog) has been related to an increased risk of numerous forms of cancer, notably colon cancer. Limiting the intake of these meats and choosing leaner protein sources, such as poultry, fish, or plant-based proteins, may be beneficial.

Moderate Alcohol Consumption: Excessive alcohol consumption is associated with an increased risk of developing several types of cancer, including liver, breast, and colorectal cancer. Limiting alcohol intake or avoiding it altogether can help reduce the risk.

Weight Management: Maintaining a healthy weight through a balanced diet and regular physical activity is important in reducing the risk of various types of cancer, including breast, colorectal, and endometrial cancer.

It's worth noting that while these dietary factors can potentially lower the risk of cancer, they should be considered as part of an overall healthy lifestyle. Other lifestyle choices such as not smoking, getting regular exercise, and avoiding exposure to environmental toxins are also essential in cancer prevention. If you have specific concerns about cancer prevention or a medical condition, it's best to consult with a healthcare professional or a registered dietitian for personalized advice.

IN WHAT WAYS CAN FOOD PREVENT CANCER

Food might prevent cancer via numerous mechanisms:

Antioxidant Protection: Many fruits, vegetables, and whole grains are high in antioxidants, such as vitamins A, C, and E, as well as phytochemicals like flavonoids and carotenoids. Antioxidants help neutralize free radicals, unstable chemicals that may harm DNA and other biological components. By lowering oxidative stress and DNA damage, antioxidants can guard against the development of cancer.

Anti-inflammatory Effects: Chronic inflammation may lead to the development of cancer. Certain foods, such as fatty fish (high in omega-3 fatty acids), nuts, seeds, and olive oil, have anti-inflammatory qualities. Including these items in your diet may help decrease inflammation in the body and perhaps minimize the risk of cancer.

Detoxification Promotes: Some foods include substances that promote the body's natural detoxification processes. Cruciferous plants like broccoli, cauliflower, and cabbage contain molecules called glucosinolates, which are transformed into active substances that help detoxify and remove toxic toxins from the body. This detoxification process may aid in minimizing the risk of cancer.

Fiber and Digestive Health: High-fiber diets, such as whole grains, legumes, fruits, and vegetables, support optimal digestive health. Fiber assists in maintaining regular bowel movements, reducing constipation, and encouraging the evacuation of waste and toxins from the body. By minimizing the exposure of the digestive system to potentially dangerous chemicals, fiber may help lessen the risk of colorectal cancer.

Hormonal Balance: Certain diets may impact hormone levels in the body, and hormonal imbalances have been related to several forms of cancer, such as breast and ovarian cancer. Consuming a diet rich in plant-based foods, such as fruits, vegetables, whole grains, and soy products, might help maintain a healthy hormonal balance and perhaps minimize the incidence of hormone-related malignancies.

Weight Management: Obesity is a risk factor for several forms of cancer. A balanced diet consisting of nutrient-dense meals, along with regular physical exercise, may help maintain a healthy weight or support weight reduction. By controlling weight, a balanced diet may minimize the incidence of obesity-related malignancies, including breast, colorectal, and endometrial cancer.

It's crucial to remember that although these pathways show how particular meals may help cancer prevention, no diet can guarantee the prevention of cancer on its own. A balanced diet, coupled with a healthy lifestyle and other preventative measures, may together help minimize the chance of acquiring cancer. It's always advisable to speak with a healthcare expert or qualified dietitian for individualized advice on nutrition and cancer prevention.

BREADS AND BREAKFAST FOODS

While there are no particular breads that may directly fight cancer, a good diet that includes certain varieties of bread can help general cancer prevention and promote a healthy lifestyle. here are some varieties of bread and nutrients that are widely regarded as healthy in the context of cancer prevention:

Whole Grain Bread: opt for bread prepared from whole grains instead of refined white flour. whole grain bread is rich in fiber, which may help maintain a healthy weight and lower the risk of some forms of cancer, such as colorectal cancer.

Sprouted Grain Bread: sprouted grain bread is created from grains that have started to germinate. It is considered to have increased nutritional content and may include beneficial substances like antioxidants, which may improve general health and perhaps lessen the incidence of some malignancies.

Bread With Seeds And Nuts: adding seeds and nuts to bread may give extra nutrients and healthy fats. flaxseeds, chia seeds, sunflower seeds, and walnuts, for example, are rich in omega-3 fatty acids and antioxidants that have been related to a decreased risk of cancer.

Bread With Vegetables: some bread variations incorporate vegetables like carrots, zucchini, or pumpkin. These additives may boost the fiber and nutritional content of the bread, leading to a healthier diet.

Remember that although including various kinds of bread in your diet might be helpful, it's crucial to concentrate on a well-rounded, plant-based diet that includes a range of fruits, vegetables, whole grains, lean proteins, and healthy fats. Additionally, speak with a healthcare practitioner or a qualified dietitian for individualized nutritional guidance, particularly if you have specific dietary needs or medical concerns.

Including cancer-fighting items in your breakfast might be a terrific way to start your day on a healthy note. here are some breakfast items that are recognized for their possible cancer-preventive properties:

Berries: blueberries, strawberries, raspberries, and other berries are rich in antioxidants, especially anthocyanins and vitamin c, which help protect cells from harm caused by free radicals. they have been related to a lower risk of numerous forms of cancer.

Whole Grain Cereals: opt for whole grain cereals such as oats, whole wheat, or bran flakes. These cereals are rich in fiber and include numerous nutrients, including antioxidants, phytochemicals, and vitamins. They may help maintain a healthy weight and minimize the risk of colorectal cancer.

Cruciferous Veggies: incorporate cruciferous vegetables like broccoli, cauliflower, kale, and brussels sprouts into your breakfast. They are rich in glucosinolates, which are substances that have been associated with a decreased risk of numerous malignancies, including lung, colorectal, and breast cancer.

Green Tea: while not a conventional morning dish, green tea may be a nutritious beverage option. It contains polyphenols, notably catechins, which have been found to have anti-cancer potential. enjoy a cup of green tea with your breakfast.

Citrus Fruits: oranges, grapefruits, lemons, and other citrus fruits are good sources of vitamin c, a potent antioxidant. vitamin c may help protect cells from harm and lessen the incidence of some malignancies, such as esophageal and stomach cancer.

Flaxseeds: sprinkle ground flaxseeds over your morning cereal or yogurt. flaxseeds are rich in omega-3 fatty acids and lignans, which have shown promise in lowering the incidence of breast and prostate cancer.

Turmeric: add a sprinkle of turmeric to your morning foods. turmeric includes an active component called curcumin, which has anti-inflammatory and antioxidant effects. It has been examined for its potential in preventing and treating numerous forms of cancer.

Remember that these foods should be part of a balanced and diverse diet. It's also vital to maintain a healthy lifestyle overall, which includes regular exercise, limiting processed foods and sugary beverages, and avoiding smoking and excessive alcohol intake. As always, contact a healthcare expert for tailored guidance, particularly if you have unique dietary requirements or medical concerns.

SAUCES, DIPS AND DRESSING

While no one sauce will guarantee the avoidance of cancer, there are specific ingredients and dietary choices that may contribute to a healthy lifestyle and may lower the chance of acquiring cancer. Here are some components typically found in sauces that are related to possible cancer-fighting properties:

Tomato-based Sauces: Tomatoes contain lycopene, a potent antioxidant that has been associated with a decreased risk of some cancers, including prostate, lung, and stomach cancers. Tomato-based sauces like marinara or salsa may be a rich source of lycopene.

Garlic Sauce: Garlic contains organosulfur chemicals that have demonstrated potential anticancer properties. These substances have been examined for their capacity to suppress the development of cancer cells and lessen the risk of specific malignancies, such as stomach, colon, and breast cancers.

Turmeric-based Sauces: Turmeric includes a chemical called curcumin, which has been intensively explored for its possible anticancer effects. Curcumin has shown promise in suppressing the proliferation of cancer cells and lowering inflammation linked with cancer development. Turmeric-based sauces, such as curry sauces, may contain curcumin.

Chili Pepper Sauce: Chili peppers contain capsaicin, a chemical that gives them their distinctive spiciness. Capsaicin has exhibited potential anticancer effects in different studies, including the capacity to trigger cell death in cancer cells and slow the development of tumors.

Olive Oil-based Sauces: Olive oil is rich in monounsaturated fats and includes numerous antioxidants, including polyphenols, which have been related to possible cancer-protective benefits. Using olive oil as a foundation for sauces may give some of these therapeutic characteristics.

It's crucial to remember that although these chemicals may have potential cancer-fighting capabilities, they are not a definite preventative or cure for cancer. A good diet, regular exercise, avoidance of cigarettes and excessive alcohol intake, and frequent cancer screenings are essential factors in minimizing the risk of cancer.

Similar to sauces, some substances are often used in dips that may have potential cancer-fighting capabilities. However, it's important to note that no single dip can guarantee the prevention of cancer. Here are some ingredients that are often found in dips and have been associated with potential cancer-protective effects:

Guacamole: Avocados, the primary ingredient in guacamole, are rich in monounsaturated fats, fiber, and various antioxidants. They also contain compounds like lutein and zeaxanthin, which have shown the potential in reducing the risk of certain cancers, such as prostate and breast cancers.

Yogurt-based Dips: Yogurt contains probiotics, which are beneficial bacteria that can promote a healthy gut microbiome. A healthy gut microbiome is associated with a reduced risk of certain types of cancer, including colorectal cancer. Opt for plain yogurt-based dips without added sugars for maximum health benefits.

Bean-based Dips: Beans, such as black beans, kidney beans, and chickpeas, are excellent sources of fiber and plant-based protein. They also contain various phytochemicals and antioxidants, including flavonoids and saponins, which have been associated with potential cancer-protective effects.

Spinach Or Kale Dips: Leafy green vegetables like spinach and kale are packed with nutrients, including vitamins, minerals, and antioxidants. These vegetables contain compounds like sulforaphane and indole-3-carbinol, which have demonstrated the potential in inhibiting the growth of cancer cells and reducing the risk of certain cancers, including lung, breast, and colorectal cancers.

Herbs And Spices: Adding herbs and spices to dips can provide additional health benefits. For example, garlic and onion contain organosulfur compounds that have shown potential anticancer effects. Turmeric, with its active compound curcumin, has also been studied for its potential cancer-fighting properties.

Remember that while incorporating these ingredients into your diet through dips may offer some potential health benefits, an overall healthy lifestyle, including a balanced diet, regular exercise, avoidance of tobacco and excessive alcohol consumption, and routine cancer screenings, is crucial for reducing the risk of cancer.

While no single food dressing can guarantee the prevention of cancer, there are certain ingredients commonly found in dressings that have been associated with potential cancer-protective effects. Here are some ingredients that are often found in dressings and have been studied for their potential health benefits:

Extra Virgin Olive Oil Dressing: Extra virgin olive oil is rich in monounsaturated fats and contains various antioxidants, such as polyphenols. These antioxidants have been associated with potential cancer-protective effects, including reducing inflammation and oxidative stress in the body. Opting for dressings made with extra virgin olive oil may provide these potential benefits.

Citrus-based Dressings: Citrus fruits like lemons, oranges, and grapefruits are rich in vitamin C and other antioxidants. Vitamin C is known for its role in immune function and can help protect cells from damage caused by free radicals. Citrus-based dressings can be a good way to incorporate these antioxidant-rich fruits into your diet.

Herb-infused Dressings: Herbs like basil, oregano, rosemary, and thyme are rich in various phytochemicals and antioxidants. These compounds have been studied for their potential anticancer effects, including inhibiting the growth of cancer cells and reducing inflammation. Using herb-infused dressings can add flavor and potentially provide some of these benefits.

Turmeric-based Dressings: Turmeric contains curcumin, a compound that has shown potential anticancer properties in various studies. Curcumin has been studied for its ability to inhibit the growth of cancer cells, reduce inflammation, and act as an antioxidant Dressings made with turmeric or curry powder may contain curcumin.

Flaxseed Oil Dressing: Flaxseed oil is a rich source of omega-3 fatty acids, lignans, and antioxidants. Omega-3 fatty acids have been connected with possible anticancer benefits, while lignans have shown promise in lowering the incidence of some hormone-related malignancies, such as breast and prostate cancers. Using flaxseed oil as a basis for dressings may give some of these possible advantages.

Remember that while incorporating these ingredients into your dressings may offer some potential health benefits, it's important to maintain an overall healthy lifestyle, including a balanced diet, regular exercise, avoidance of tobacco and excessive alcohol consumption, and routine cancer screenings, to reduce the risk of cancer.

SIDES AND VEGGIES

While no one meal or side dish will ensure the prevention of cancer, several food choices have been connected with possible cancer-protective benefits when consumed as part of a healthy, balanced diet. Here are several meal sides that are renowned for their possible health benefits:

Cruciferous Vegetables: Vegetables such as broccoli, cauliflower, Brussels sprouts, kale, and cabbage belong to the cruciferous family. They are rich in fiber, vitamins, minerals, and phytochemicals. Cruciferous vegetables include substances including sulforaphane and indole-3-carbinol, which have been researched for their ability to prevent cancer cell proliferation and lower the incidence of several cancers, including lung, colorectal, and breast cancers.

Leafy Greens: Leafy greens like spinach, kale, Swiss chard, and arugula are filled with nutrients, including vitamins, minerals, and antioxidants. They are high in fiber and contain several phytochemicals that have been related to possible cancer-protective properties. Regularly including leafy greens in your diet may contribute to general health and may help lessen the risk of some malignancies.

Colorful Fruits And Vegetables: Fruits and vegetables of varied hues, such as berries, tomatoes, carrots, bell peppers, and sweet potatoes, contain a range of antioxidants, vitamins, and minerals. These nutrients assist sustain a healthy immune system and protect cells from harm. Including a variety of colored fruits and vegetables in your meals may give a range of possible health advantages, including potential cancer prevention.

Legumes: Legumes, including beans, lentils, and chickpeas, are good sources of fiber, plant-based protein, vitamins, and minerals.

They also include phytochemicals and antioxidants. Regular eating of beans has been connected with a lower risk of some malignancies, such as colorectal cancer. Incorporating beans as a side dish or in salads may be a healthful addition to your meals.

Whole Grains: Whole grains like brown rice, quinoa, whole wheat, oats, and barley are rich in fiber, vitamins, minerals, and antioxidants. They offer more nutritional value compared to refined grains. Whole grains have been associated with a reduced risk of various types of cancer, including colorectal cancer. Opting for whole-grain side dishes instead of refined grains can be a healthier choice.

Remember that a well-balanced diet, coupled with a healthy lifestyle that includes regular exercise, avoidance of tobacco and excessive alcohol intake, and frequent cancer screenings, is crucial to minimizing the risk of cancer. These food sides may be part of a balanced diet, but they should be coupled with other healthy options for the best benefits.

Several vegetables have been examined for their possible cancer-fighting qualities owing to their substantial nutritional content and bioactive chemicals. Including these veggies in your diet may help to a healthy lifestyle and perhaps lessen the risk of some malignancies. Here are several veggies that have shown potential in combating cancer:

Tomatoes: Tomatoes are a good source of vitamins (such as vitamin C and vitamin A), minerals, and antioxidants. They also contain lycopene, a strong antioxidant that has been intensively examined for its possible cancer-fighting qualities. Lycopene has shown promise in lowering the risk of numerous malignancies, including prostate, lung, and stomach cancers. Cooking tomatoes or ingesting them with a source of fat (like olive oil) might boost the absorption of lycopene.

Carrots: Carrots are rich in beta-carotene, a precursor of vitamin A, as well as other antioxidants and dietary fiber. Beta-carotene is renowned for its capacity to serve as an antioxidant and protect cells from harm. Carrots have been connected with a lower risk of numerous malignancies, including lung, colorectal, and stomach cancers.

Garlic And Onions: Garlic and onions belong to the Allium family of plants and contain organosulfur compounds, including allicin and diallyl sulfide, which have been researched for their possible anticancer effects. These chemicals have shown the capacity to block cancer cell proliferation and lower the risk of numerous malignancies, including stomach, colorectal, and prostate cancers.

Remember, although these veggies may provide possible cancer-fighting advantages, it's vital to maintain a well-rounded diet that includes a mix of fruits, vegetables, whole grains, lean proteins, and healthy fats. Additionally, adopting other healthy lifestyle habits, such as regular exercise, avoiding cigarettes and excessive alcohol intake, and frequent cancer screenings, is vital for minimizing the risk of cancer.

SOUPS AND SALADS

While no one soup will guarantee the prevention or treatment of cancer, integrating specific nutrients in soups might contribute to a balanced diet and perhaps give cancer-fighting effects. Here are some substances often present in soups that have been related to possible cancer-protective effects:

Vegetable-based Soups: Soups cooked largely with a variety of vegetables may be a fantastic way to add cancer-fighting nutrients to your diet. Vegetables including cruciferous vegetables (broccoli, cauliflower, kale), leafy greens (spinach, Swiss chard), tomatoes, carrots, onions, garlic, and mushrooms are rich in vitamins, minerals, antioxidants, and phytochemicals that have been researched for their possible cancer-fighting effects.

Turmeric-based Soups: Turmeric includes curcumin, a substance that has proven possible anticancer properties. Including turmeric in your soups, such as in curries or lentil soups, may give some of the possible health advantages associated with curcumin, including its anti-inflammatory and antioxidant qualities.

Legume-based Soups: Soups cooked with legumes like lentils, chickpeas, and beans are good sources of fiber, plant-based protein, vitamins, minerals, and phytonutrients. Legumes contain numerous chemicals, including flavonoids and lignans, which have shown promise in lowering the risk of some malignancies, such as colorectal, breast, and prostate cancers.

Mushroom Soups: Certain mushrooms, such as shiitake, maitake, and reishi, have been examined for their possible anticancer properties. They include substances such as polysaccharides, beta-glucans, and triterpenes that have shown promise in boosting the immune system, preventing cancer cell development, and lowering inflammation. Including mushroom-based soups in your diet may give some of these possible advantages.

Bone Broth-based Soups: Bone broth, created by boiling bones and connective tissues, may supply critical nutrients and minerals. It is typically used as a basis for soups. While further study is required, bone broth may improve general health by supplying collagen, amino acids, and minerals that are helpful for the body. It may also assist maintain gut health, which plays a part in the overall immunological function.

Remember, a healthy diet should be well-rounded and contain a range of foods. It's vital to combine these cancer-fighting elements with other healthy lifestyle choices, including regular exercise, avoidance of cigarettes and excessive alcohol intake, and frequent cancer screenings, to minimize the risk of cancer and preserve general well-being.

Including certain items in your salads might give anti-cancer advantages owing to their high nutritional value and possible cancer-fighting capabilities. It's essential to emphasize that although a nutritious diet might help general well-being, it's not a replacement for medical advice or treatment. Here are some foods you might try incorporating into your salads that have been related to possible anti-cancer properties:

Colorful Veggies: Include a range of colorful vegetables such as bell peppers, tomatoes, carrots, beets, and radishes. These veggies include a spectrum of antioxidants, vitamins, and minerals that help promote a healthy immune system and general well-being.

Berries: Berries including strawberries, blueberries, raspberries, and blackberries are high in antioxidants, notably anthocyanins.

These chemicals have been connected with anti-cancer properties and may help decrease inflammation.

Nuts And Seeds: Add a sprinkling of nuts and seeds such as walnuts, almonds, flaxseeds, and chia seeds to your salad. They supply healthful fats and include phytochemicals such as lignans that have potential anti-cancer qualities.

Citrus Fruits: Citrus fruits like oranges, lemons, and grapefruits are strong in vitamin C and other antioxidants. Vitamin C is known to support a healthy immune system and may help reduce the risk of certain cancers.

Garlic And Onions: Both garlic and onions contain sulfur compounds that have been associated with potential cancer-fighting properties. They can be used in dressings or as flavorful additions to your salad.

Remember, a balanced and varied diet is essential for overall health, and it's always a good idea to consult with a healthcare professional or a registered dietitian for personalized advice, especially if you have specific dietary concerns or medical conditions.

BEVERAGES

While it's crucial to remember that no one beverage can promise to prevent or cure cancer, some drinks may contain substances that have been investigated for their possible cancer-fighting capabilities. Including these drinks as part of a balanced and nutritious diet may help overall well-being. Here are several drinks that have been related to possible cancer-fighting properties:

Green Tea: Green tea includes polyphenols, notably catechins, which have been researched for their possible anti-cancer properties. These chemicals have shown promise in laboratory experiments by helping to prevent the development of cancer cells and minimize tumor formation. However, additional study is required to grasp the full range of green tea's advantages.

Turmeric Tea: Turmeric includes an active chemical called curcumin, which exhibits significant anti-inflammatory and antioxidant effects. Curcumin has been examined for its ability to suppress the development of cancer cells and decrease inflammation in the body. Turmeric tea, produced by steeping turmeric powder or grated turmeric root in hot water, may be a method to add this healthful spice into your diet.

Pomegranate Juice: Pomegranates are rich in antioxidants, especially polyphenols, which may help decrease oxidative stress and inflammation in the body. Some research has shown that pomegranate extract or juice may have potential anti-cancer benefits, notably against breast and prostate cancer. However, additional study is required to discover the full range of its advantages.

Tomato Juice: Tomatoes contain a potent antioxidant called lycopene, which gives them their brilliant red color. Lycopene has been examined for its ability to lessen the risk of various malignancies, such as prostate, lung, and stomach cancers. Tomato juice is a handy method to absorb lycopene since the heating process helps to release and boost its absorption.

Beetroot Juice: Beets are rich in minerals and phytochemicals, including betalains, which are responsible for their deep red color. Betalains exhibit antioxidant and anti-inflammatory characteristics and have been researched for their possible anti-cancer benefits. While research is continuing, beetroot juice may be a useful complement to a balanced diet.

Remember that the entire food pattern is vital for cancer prevention. It's crucial to eat a mix of fruits, vegetables, whole grains, lean proteins, and healthy fats while keeping a balanced and active lifestyle. It's always advisable to speak with a healthcare expert or a qualified dietitian for specialized advice about your health requirements.

SMOOTHIES

Smoothies can be a superb way to incorporate cancer-preventing ingredients into your diet. While it is important to note that no single food or smoothie can warranty the prevention of cancer, sure components have been related to doable cancer-fighting properties. Here are some kinds of smoothies that can consist of such ingredients:

1. Berry Blast Smoothie:

Ingredients: Blueberries, strawberries, raspberries, spinach, almond milk, chia seeds. Blueberries and raspberries are rich in antioxidants, which may help combat free radicals that can contribute to most cancers' development. Spinach is packed with vitamins and minerals, while chia seeds furnish omega-3 fatty acids, fiber, and protein.

2. Green Power Smoothie:

Ingredients: Kale, spinach, cucumber, green apple, ginger, lemon juice, coconut water.

Kale and spinach are leafy veggies that are excessive in antioxidants and nutrients. Cucumber offers hydration and contributes to detoxification. Ginger has anti-inflammatory properties, and lemon juice adds a fresh twist. Coconut water offers electrolytes and hydration.

3. Turmeric Tropical Smoothie:

Ingredients: Pineapple, mango, turmeric, coconut milk, Greek yogurt, honey.

Turmeric includes curcumin, a compound with anti-inflammatory and viable anti-cancer properties. Pineapple and mango supply imperative vitamins and minerals, while coconut milk and Greek yogurt add creaminess. Honey can be used as a herbal sweetener.

4. Cruciferous Veggie Smoothie:

Ingredients: Kale, broccoli, cauliflower, inexperienced apple, pear, almond milk, flaxseeds.

Cruciferous vegetables like kale, broccoli, and cauliflower incorporate sulforaphane and other compounds that have shown achievable in most cancer prevention. Green apple and pear add natural sweetness and fiber, whilst almond milk and flax seeds provide wholesome fat and extra nutrients.

Remember, these smoothies should be part of a balanced and diverse weight-reduction plan that includes a large variety of fruits, vegetables, complete grains, lean proteins, and wholesome fats. It's continually an excellent concept to consult with a healthcare professional or registered dietitian for personalized dietary hints related to cancer prevention.

DESSERT

While no one dessert may conclusively treat cancer, you can prepare sweets with foods that are connected with possible cancer-fighting effects. Here's a dessert suggestion utilizing some of these ingredients:

Recipe: Mixed Berry Chia Seed Pudding

Ingredients:

- 1 cup mixed berries (blueberries, raspberries, strawberries)
- 2 teaspoons chia seeds
- 1 cup almond milk (or other plant-based milk)
- 1 tablespoon honey or maple syrup (optional)
- A sprinkling of dark chocolate shavings (70% cocoa or higher)
- A pinch of turmeric powder (optional)

Instructions:

- In a blender, puree the mixed berries until smooth.
- In a dish, add the blended berries, chia seeds, almond milk, and sweetener (if preferred). Stir well to mix.
- Let the mixture rest for approximately 5 minutes to enable the chia seeds to absorb the liquid. Stir again to avoid clumping.
- Cover the bowl and refrigerate for at least 2 hours or overnight, until the mixture thickens and produces a pudding-like consistency.
- Once cooled and thickened, divide the pudding into serving dishes or glasses.
- Top each dish with a sprinkle of dark chocolate shavings and a sprinkling of turmeric powder for extra taste and possible health benefits.
- Serve and enjoy your mixed berry chia seed pudding as a delightful and perhaps healthful dessert choice.

Remember, although including cancer-fighting elements into your desserts is a great beginning, it's crucial to maintain an overall healthy and balanced diet, exercise frequently, and speak with a healthcare expert for customized guidance on cancer prevention and treatment.

RECIPES FOR PREVENTION

Smoothies can be a superb way to incorporate cancer-preventing ingredients into your diet. While it is important to note that no single food or smoothie can warranty the prevention of cancer, sure components have been related to doable cancer-fighting properties. Here are some kinds of smoothies that can consist of such ingredients:

1. Berry Blast Smoothie:

Ingredients: Blueberries, strawberries, raspberries, spinach, almond milk, chia seeds.
Blueberries and raspberries are rich in antioxidants, which may help combat free radicals that can contribute to most cancers' development. Spinach is packed with vitamins and minerals, while chia seeds furnish omega-3 fatty acids, fiber, and protein.

2. Green Power Smoothie:

Ingredients: Kale, spinach, cucumber, green apple, ginger, lemon juice, coconut water.
Kale and spinach are leafy veggies that are excessive in antioxidants and nutrients. Cucumber offers hydration and contributes to detoxification. Ginger has anti-inflammatory properties, and lemon juice adds a fresh twist. Coconut water offers electrolytes and hydration.

2. Turmeric Tropical Smoothie:

Ingredients: Pineapple, mango, turmeric, coconut milk, Greek yogurt, honey.
Turmeric includes curcumin, a compound with anti-inflammatory and viable anti-cancer properties. Pineapple and mango supply imperative vitamins and minerals, while coconut milk and Greek yogurt add creaminess. Honey can be used as a herbal sweetener.

3. Cruciferous Veggie Smoothie:

Ingredients: Kale, broccoli, cauliflower, inexperienced apple, pear, almond milk, flaxseeds.

Cruciferous vegetables like kale, broccoli, and cauliflower incorporate sulforaphane and other compounds that have shown achievable in most cancer prevention. Green apple and pear add natural sweetness and fiber, whilst almond milk and flax seeds provide wholesome fat and extra nutrients.

Remember, these smoothies should be part of a balanced and diverse weight-reduction plan that includes a large variety of fruits, vegetables, complete grains, lean proteins, and wholesome fats. It's continually an excellent concept to consult with a healthcare professional or registered dietitian for personalized dietary hints related to cancer prevention.

RECIPES FOR THOSE RECEIVING CANCER TREATMENT

When presenting the process of most cancer treatments, it is important to hold a well-balanced food regimen that presents fundamental nutrients and helps typical health. Here are a few recipe ideas that are nutritious and effortless to prepare:

1. Creamy Vegetable Soup:

Ingredients: Assorted vegetables (carrots, broccoli, cauliflower, zucchini, etc.), low-sodium vegetable broth, low-fat milk or non-dairy milk, garlic, onion, herbs (such as thyme or basil), salt, and pepper.

Instructions: Sauté garlic and onion in a pot, add chopped vegetables and cook till tender. Add vegetable broth and herbs, then simmer until veggies are soft. Blend the combination until smooth, then add milk, salt, and pepper to taste. Heat the soup until heated and served.

2. Baked Salmon with Quinoa and Roasted Vegetables:

Ingredients: Fresh salmon filets, quinoa, combined veggies (such as bell peppers, Brussels sprouts, and sweet potatoes), olive oil, lemon juice, garlic, salt, and pepper.

Instructions: Preheat the oven to 375°F (190°C). Season the salmon filets with olive oil, lemon juice, minced garlic, salt, and pepper. Place them on a baking sheet and bake for 15-20 minutes till cooked through. Cook quinoa in accordance to bundle instructions. Toss the combined veggies with olive oil, salt, and pepper, then roast in the oven for 20-25 minutes. Serve the salmon over quinoa with roasted greens on the side.

Quinoa And Black Bean Salad:

Ingredients: Cooked quinoa, canned black beans (rinsed and drained), cherry tomatoes (halved), cucumber (diced), purple onion (finely chopped), fresh cilantro (chopped), lime juice, olive oil, salt, and pepper.

Instructions: In a bowl, mix quinoa, black beans, cherry tomatoes, cucumber, red onion, and cilantro. In a separate small bowl, whisk together lime juice, olive oil, salt, and pepper to make the dressing. Pour the dressing over the quinoa combination and toss nicely to combine. Refrigerate for at least 30 minutes earlier than serving.

Berry And Spinach Smoothie:

Ingredients: Fresh or frozen berries (strawberries, blueberries, raspberries), clean spinach leaves, Greek yogurt (or dairy-free alternative), almond milk (or desired milk), honey (optional), and ice cubes.

Instructions: Place berries, spinach, Greek yogurt, almond milk, honey (if desired), and ice cubes in a blender. Blend till smooth and creamy. Adjust the consistency with the aid of including extra almond milk if needed. Serve chilled.

Remember, it is important to personalize your diet based totally on your unique dietary desires and any dietary restrictions you might also have. Consult with a registered dietitian or a healthcare expert who specializes in oncology for individualized recommendations and recommendations.

FOODS TO AVOID WHEN FIGHTING CANCER

When combating cancer, it is crucial to keep a healthy and balanced diet. While no one meal can guarantee the prevention or cure of cancer, some dietary choices may improve general health and perhaps lessen the chance of acquiring cancer or its development. Here are some basic tips on foods to restrict or avoid while treating cancer:

Processed And Cured Foods: Consumption of processed meats including hot dogs, bacon, sausages, and deli meats has been related to an increased risk of cancer, especially colorectal cancer. These meats frequently include preservatives, chemicals, and excessive quantities of salt.

Red Meat: High intake of red meat, such as beef, hog, and lamb, has been connected with an elevated risk of numerous forms of cancer, including colorectal, pancreatic, and prostate cancer. If you prefer to consume red meat, choose lean cuts and minimize the quantity size.

Sugar And Sugary Foods: A diet heavy in added sugars and sugary foods may lead to obesity and inflammation, which are risk factors for different malignancies. Limit your consumption of sugary beverages, desserts, sweets, and processed foods.

Refined Grains And White Flour Products: Refined grains have had their bran and germ removed, resulting in a loss of fiber, vitamins, and minerals. Examples include white bread, white rice, and pasta made from refined flour. These foods may produce rises in blood sugar levels and may trigger inflammation.

Trans Fats And Bad Fats: Trans fats are present in many processed and fried meals, such as professionally baked items, packaged snacks, and fast food. These fats may induce inflammation and raise the risk of many malignancies. Choose healthy fats like olive oil, avocado, almonds, and seeds.

Alcohol: Excessive alcohol intake has been associated with an increased risk of various forms of cancer, including breast, liver, and colorectal cancer. It is suggested to minimize or avoid alcohol completely, especially if you are receiving cancer treatment.

Excessive Salt: High-sodium diets have been related to an increased risk of stomach cancer. Limit your consumption of processed meals, canned items, and fast food, which generally include excessive quantities of salt.

Remember, it is vital to contact a healthcare practitioner or a registered dietitian who specializes in oncology for individualized dietary recommendations based on your unique health condition, treatment plan, and individual requirements. They may give counsel customized to your circumstances and ensure

that your diet promotes your general well-being
throughout cancer treatment.

CONCLUSION

While there is no surefire method to prevent cancer purely via nutrition, a healthy and balanced diet may help lower the chance of acquiring some forms of cancer. Here are some eating suggestions that are connected with cancer prevention:

Cruciferous Vegetables: Broccoli, cauliflower, Brussels sprouts, kale, and cabbage are high in antioxidants and contain substances that have been related to a decreased risk of several cancers, including lung, colorectal, breast, and prostate cancers.

Berries: Blueberries, strawberries, raspberries, and blackberries are filled with antioxidants and phytochemicals that have been demonstrated to have anti-cancer qualities. They may help reduce inflammation and protect against several forms of cancer, including colon, breast, and prostate cancer.

Garlic: Garlic contains sulfur compounds that have been related to a decreased incidence of stomach, colon, and esophageal cancers. It may also assist improve the immune system and have anti-inflammatory properties.

Tomatoes: Tomatoes are a rich source of lycopene, an antioxidant that gives them their brilliant red color. Lycopene has been related to a decreased incidence of prostate, lung, and stomach cancers. Cooking tomatoes and using them with a little oil might boost the absorption of lycopene.

Green Tea: Green tea is high in antioxidants known as catechins. Regular drinking of green tea has been connected with a lower risk of numerous forms of cancer, including breast, prostate, and colorectal cancers.

Turmeric: Curcumin, the main ingredient in turmeric, has potent anti-inflammatory and antioxidant effects. It has shown promise in slowing the proliferation of cancer cells and avoiding the creation of tumors, notably in colorectal, breast, and prostate malignancies.

Fish: Fatty fish such as salmon, mackerel, and sardines are great providers of omega-3 fatty acids. Omega-3s have been associated with a decreased incidence of colon, prostate, and breast malignancies. Aim for two servings of fish every week.

Leafy Greens: Spinach, kale, Swiss chard, and other leafy greens are filled with vitamins, minerals, and antioxidants. They are helpful for general health and have been related to a lower risk of various forms of cancer, including lung, breast, and colorectal cancers.

Nuts And Seeds: Almonds, walnuts, flaxseeds, and chia seeds are rich in fiber, healthy fats, and antioxidants. They have been related to a decreased incidence of colorectal, breast, and prostate cancers.

Whole Grains: Whole grains including brown rice, quinoa, oats, and whole wheat include fiber, vitamins, minerals, and phytochemicals that may help lower the risk of different malignancies, notably colon cancer.

Remember, it's crucial to have a healthy lifestyle overall, including regular exercise, limiting processed foods and added sugars, avoiding excessive alcohol use, and not smoking, since these variables also play a key influence in cancer prevention.

www.ingramcontent.com/pod-product-compliance
Lightning Source LLC
Chambersburg PA
CBHW070501220526
45466CB00004B/1922